MW01030773

BIBLE CURE ®

FOR

PMS AND MOOD SWINGS

DON COLBERT, M.D.

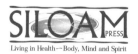

Living in Health--Body, Mind and Spirit

THE BIBLE CURE FOR PMS AND MOOD SWINGS
by Don Colbert, M.D.
Published by Siloam Press
A part of Strang Communications Company
600 Rinehart Road
Lake Mary, Florida 32746
www.siloampress.com

Library of Congress Catalog Card Number: 00-112294
International Standard Book Number: 0-88419-745-X

This book is not intended to provide medical advice or to take the place of medical advice and treatment from your personal physician. Readers are advised to consult their own doctors or other qualified health professionals regarding the treatment of their medical problems. Neither the publisher nor the author takes any responsibility for any possible consequences from any treatment, action or application of medicine, supplement, herb or preparation to any person reading or following the information in this book. If readers are taking prescription medications, they should consult with their physicians and not take themselves off of medicines to start supplementation without the proper supervision of a physician.

01 02 03 04 05 9 8 7 6 5 4
Printed in the United States of America

Discover the Truth About PMS

If you believe that PMS is a miserable curse that you must accept, then you have believed a lie. The truth about PMS is that God never intended for you to feel absolutely miserable—not even for one minute!

The Bible says, "For the LORD takes pleasure in His people; He will beautify the afflicted ones with salvation" (Ps. 149:4, NAS).

If you have been suffering from the pain and discomfort of PMS every month, I have good news for you. You can begin to put those depressing days of pain and discomfort behind you.

The Bible says, "He has sent me to tell those who mourn that the time of the LORD's favor has come, and with it, the day of God's anger against their enemies. To all who mourn in Israel, he will give beauty for ashes, joy instead of mourning, praise instead of despair. For the Lord has planted them like strong and graceful oaks for his own glory" (Isa. 61:2–3).

The notion that you must simply endure discomfort and pain is nothing more than an old wives' tale. God desires for you to feel great every day of your life. This book will empower you to take charge of your PMS symptoms. It is power-packed with important information about nutrition, lifestyle, supplements and many other natural methods to combat the monthly symptoms of PMS. More importantly, this booklet is charged with dynamic truth from God's Word that will recharge your spirit, renew your mind and strengthen your faith.

PMS

If you've ever suffered with PMS, you're already painfully aware of those uncomfortable symptoms every seven to fourteen days before your cycle begins: irritability, decreased sex drive, headache, breast pain, abdominal bloating, stress and tension, fatigue, mood swings, depression, backache and swelling in fingers, feet and ankles.

About one-third of all women suffer with PMS, and as many as 5 percent of all women experience severe PMS.

Premenopause, on the other hand, is an assortment of symptoms in women and occurs about ten to twenty years before menopause, usually when a woman is between ages thirty and fifty. Common symptoms include PMS; weight gain; fatigue; irritability; mood swings and depression; tender, enlarged or lumpy breasts; uterine fibroids; endometriosis; migraine headaches; loss of memory; menstrual irregularities, including bleeding between periods, very light periods or very heavy periods; problems conceiving and cold hands and feet.

But these symptoms do not have to happen to you!

A Bold, New Approach

With the help of the practical and faith-inspiring wisdom contained in this Bible Cure booklet, you can rise above the discomfort of PMS. Not only that, but many individuals who experience even severe PMS discomfort can live free of the symptoms completely. Through the power of good nutrition, healthy lifestyle choices, exercise, vitamins and supplements, and most importantly of all, through the power of dynamic faith, you can be empowered to halt the debilitating symptoms of PMS.

PMS is not something you have to accept. With God's grace, mental accuracy, power and increasing joy await you.

As you read this book, prepare to win the battle against PMS. In this Bible Cure booklet, filled with practical steps, hope, encouragement and valuable information on how to develop a healthy, empowered lifestyle, you will

uncover God's divine plan of health
for body, soul and spirit
through modern medicine, good nutrition
and the medicinal power
of Scripture and prayer.

You will also discover life-changing scriptures throughout this booklet that will strengthen and encourage you.

As you read, apply and trust God's promises, you will also uncover powerful Bible Cure prayers to help you line up your thoughts and feelings with God's plan of divine health for you—a plan that includes living victoriously. In this Bible Cure booklet, you will discover powerful insight in the following chapters:

You can confidently take the natural and spiritual steps outlined in this book to overcome PMS forever.

It is my prayer that these practical suggestions for health, nutrition and fitness will bring wholeness to your life—body, soul and spirit. May they deepen your fellowship with God and strengthen your ability to worship and serve Him.

—DON COLBERT, M.D.

A BIBLE CURE PRAYER
FOR YOU

Dear God, I pray that You take the veil off of the eyes of each precious person who reads this book. Let Your daughters know with great certainty that You never intended for them to suffer with monthly pain and discomfort. Reveal Your heart of love, and teach Your people that You are indeed their healer. Amen.

Chapter 1

Truth That
Sets You Free

The Bible says, "And you will know the truth, and the truth will set you free" (John 8:32). Now you may never have considered that this scripture included PMS, but it does. It concerns all truth—even the truth about your body and your health!

Believing a lie can bring you into bondage and can cause you to passively accept circumstances or situations that you should never accept. For example, if you were told that you were created by God to be poor and broke, you might accept poverty. If your boss refused to pay you, you might accept that as your lot in life without even resisting. If thieves and robbers stole your goods, you might not even attempt to fight back. That acceptance would be created by the lie that caused you to allow poverty into your life in a way

1

in which God never intended.

It works the same with your health. If you believe that the monthly discomfort of PMS is your lot in life as a woman, that belief system could then cause you to passively accept what God never intended rather than searching for a cure. It's my desire that you really know the heart of God toward you.

God has not cursed you. As a matter of fact, He has spoken great and powerful blessings over your life. Here are a few:

> All these blessings shall overtake you, if you will obey the LORD your God. Blessed shall you be in the city, and blessed shall you be in the country. Blessed shall be the offspring of your body and the produce of your ground and the offspring of your beasts, the increase of your herd and the young of your flock. Blessed shall be your basket and your kneading bowl. Blessed shall you be when you come in, and blessed shall you be when you go out.
>
> The LORD will cause your enemies who rise up against you to be defeated before you; they shall come out against

you one way and shall flee before you seven ways. The LORD will command the blessing upon you in your barns and in all that you put your hand to, and He will bless you in the land which the LORD your God gives you . . . And the LORD will make you abound in prosperity, in the offspring of your body and in the offspring of your beast and in the produce of your ground.

—DEUTERONOMY 28:2–8, 11, NAS

Even in the face of all these powerful blessings, some might say, "Well, these blessings were for Israel, not for me." You are wrong! The Bible says that Christ died "in order that in Christ Jesus the blessing of Abraham might come to the Gentiles" (Gal. 3:14, NAS).

God has richly blessed you! You are richly, powerfully and wonderfully blessed!

You Are God's Masterpiece!

While you're experiencing PMS it might be difficult to think of your body as being especially blessed, but it is. With supernatural genius, God created your body as a living masterpiece—a divinely engineered work of art. And with just a little bit of God's wisdom, you can learn to work with your body to help it function better so that you will truly feel better.

To understand PMS and premenopause, it is important to have a good basic understanding of what is happening in your body. Let's look.

> *May God pass on to you and your descendants the blessings he promised to Abraham.*
> —GENESIS 28:4

Your Incredible Body

Your incredible body is far more complex and more wonderful than any machine ever made. At birth, a baby girl has about seven hundred thousand eggs in her ovaries. By the time she reaches puberty, many of these eggs dissolve, leaving only four hundred thousand. Even so, this young woman will only experience about four hundred to five hundred ovulations in her lifetime when an egg is actually released from an ovary.

No doubt you're familiar with the hormone estrogen. Actually it's only one of many hormones involved in this incredible process. When a young girl begins her monthly menstrual cycle, her body begins releasing and orchestrating an intricate symphony of many different powerful hormones. These hormones are the catalyst for everything that takes place. Let's take a brief look at these different hormones.

The hypothalamus, the pituitary gland and the ovaries release these powerful hormones. The hormone GnRH (or gonadotropin-releasing hormone) triggers the release of hormones from the pituitary gland. GnRH then triggers the pituitary gland to secrete two hormones that cause the egg to mature and eventually to be released from the ovaries.

Shortly after a woman starts her period, the pituitary gland begins to release FSH (or follicle-stimulating hormone). FSH stimulates the growth of about six to twelve eggs and their sacs, called follicles, in the ovaries. Only one egg will fully mature and be released from the ovary. The other eggs and their sacs will then dissolve.

At about day fourteen of the menstrual cycle, which is usually right in the middle, the pituitary gland releases another hormone called LH, or luteinizing hormone. This hormone causes the follicle to swell and rupture, releasing the egg from the ovary, which is called ovulation.

However, prior to the release of the egg

estrogen levels increase. Estrogen causes the lining of the uterus to thicken to prepare to receive the egg.

After the ruptured follicle has released its egg, the cells lining the ruptured follicle form the corpus luteum, which secretes the hormone progesterone. This progesterone signals the lining of the

> *He will love you and bless you and make you into a great nation. He will give you many children and give fertility to your land and you animals.*
> —DEUTERONOMY 7:13

uterus to thicken even more. As estrogen and other related hormone levels rise, a signal is then sent to the pituitary gland to stop producing LH and FSH. When these hormones decrease, the corpus luteum begins to degenerate, which signals a drop of both estrogen and progesterone.

When these two hormone levels drop, the lining of the uterus sloughs off and menstruation begins.

This is not the end, however. The symphony plays on as the pituitary gland once again begins to secrete FSH and LH, which again stimulates more follicles to be developed. Now the entire cycle begins all over again. So you have it, the marvelous and masterful process that allows your body to bring to birth a living being—procreated from the very image of God. Amazing!

Supporting Your
Body's Delicate Balance

This intricate interplay of hormones within your cycle is properly orchestrated by three players: the hypothalamus, the pituitary gland and the ovaries.

It's vital that these players produce and secrete the necessary hormones at just the right time in your cycle. This delicate balance of hormones can be upset by many different factors.

All steroid hormones, which include progesterone and estrogen, are first manufactured from cholesterol. Cholesterol, as you know, comes from your diet.

We have learned that cholesterol is the enemy—but it actually forms the foundation of all steroid sex hormones. Therefore, a small amount of cholesterol or saturated fat in the diet is necessary for hormonal balance.

Cholesterol is converted to pregnenolone, and pregnenolone is eventually converted to progesterone and estrogen. Many steps take place along the way. But if your body lacks the raw materials for this process, it can't make sufficient amounts of hormones. Without enough of the right ingredients, the outcome will doubtless be affected—and your body's delicate hormonal balance will be thrown off.

Those raw materials include cholesterol, specific vitamins, minerals and enzymes—especially magnesium and vitamin B_6

Too much stress can also throw off your hormonal balance as well. Stress causes excessive amounts of cortisol to be released into your bloodstream. As your cortisol levels rise, your body will begin to demand more and more progesterone. That's because cortisol is actually made from progesterone. This also leads to symptoms of PMS.

You May Not Be Ovulating

Even though they may be completely unaware of it, many women have stopped ovulating even though they continue to have regular monthly periods.

If a woman doesn't ovulate, her body misses a beat and the hormonal balance is disrupted. It would be like trying to play a musical score without a major instrument—the orchestration drops a beat, and instead of producing soothing music, the entire symphony begins to screech and squawk.

When you don't ovulate, the corpus luteum is not formed. The corpus luteum is responsible for secreting large amounts of progesterone—so you end up without enough progesterone.

Here are some factors that can cause you to stop ovulating:

- Too much stress
- Poor nutrition
- Exposure to xeno-hormones or xeno-estrogens, which are man-made chemicals with hormonal effects
- Inadequate amounts of the necessary vitamins, minerals and enzymes to convert one hormone to another

Let's look at some of these factors. Are you . . .

Out of balance?

If you have too much or too little estrogen, testosterone, cortisol, progesterone or any of the intermediate hormones, such as pregnenolone and DHEA, it's easy to see how your body's delicate balance could be disrupted.

Too active?

Although it's not a problem for most of us, too much physical exercise can be as detrimental as too little. The rigorous physical lifestyles of some female athletes, such as long-distance runners, can cause them to stop ovulating.

Too busy?

Excessive mental stress works the same way. In our fast-paced society, many women shoulder so many responsibilities, such as full-time employment, taxi driver for the kids, full-time cook, laundry and cleaning lady, Cub Scout mom—and the list goes on and on. There simply aren't enough hours in a day for all activities that many women attempt to do. Before long you find yourself cutting into your sleep schedule—and your rest becomes seriously compromised.

> *May God Almighty bless you and give you many children. And may your descendants become a great assembly of nations.*
> —GENESIS 28:3

Over time, the rigors of such lifestyles take a real toll upon a woman's mind and body. One result is the cessation of ovulation. Your PMS symptoms could actually be your body's way of signaling you to take it a little slower. We'll look more at this later.

This excessive stress is commonly associated with anovulatory cycles in which a woman doesn't ovulate and, thus, doesn't produce enough progesterone.

Too emotionally wrung out?

Emotional stress can also do the same. The death of a loved one, a divorce, dealing with a child with ADD, dealing with children on drugs, anxiety and depression can also cause excessive stress, resulting in anovulatory cycles.

Let's take a closer look at each of these powerful hormones and why they are so important to your health.

Estrogen and Your Body

You may be surprised to learn there is more than one type of estrogen. Actually, including plant-made estrogens and man-made varieties, there are several:

- Estradiol, which is produced in the ovaries

- Estrone, which is produced in fatty tissues

- Estriol, which is produced primarily in the adrenal glands

- Xeno-estrogens, which are environmental

chemicals that work like estrogens in your body

- Phytoestrogens, which are plant compounds with weak, estrogen-like effects

- Synthetic estrogen, which is used in hormone replacement therapy and birth control pills

In a manner of speaking, estrogen is actually what makes a girl a woman. This mighty hormone estrogen is key in a little girl's development of sexual characteristics including the breasts, pubic hair and female sex organs. Estrogen is also critical in pregnancy and in maintaining the menstrual cycle. It is estrogen that stimulates the lining of the uterus to grow, preparing a woman's body for pregnancy.

Estrogen stimulates cell growth, and too much estrogen can actually be a promoter for cancer of the breast, uterus and ovaries. That's where progesterone comes in. Progesterone helps to prevent cancer by balancing the hormones and minimizing the growth properties of estrogen.

Is Your Body Making Too Much?

Estrogen dominance was actually brought to light

by renowned physician Dr. John Lee.[1] Estrogen dominance is simply excess estrogen that has not been balanced by progesterone. Estrogen dominance is very common in the U.S. and accounts for many of the symptoms of premenopause.

Xeno is Greek for *alien,* or *stranger.* Estrogen dominance is often caused by xeno-hormones, or xeno-estrogens, which are man-made chemicals in the environment that fool your body into believing they are natural estrogen. Your bloodstream invites these strangers in, just like a Trojan horse, where they begin to throw your entire hormonal system out of balance. Xeno-estrogens bind to estrogen receptors and can predispose you to estrogen dominance, premenopausal symptoms and even cancer.

Since most xeno-estrogens are non-biodegradable, as you get older they tend to become increasingly concentrated in your fatty tissues. This could be one of the main

> *Harmony is as refreshing as the dew from Mount Hermon that falls on the mountains of Zion. And the* Lord *has pronounced his blessing, even life forevermore.*
> —Psalm 133:3

reasons that we are seeing an increase in both prostate and breast cancer due to ever-increasing exposure to xeno-estrogens.

In the book *Our Stolen Future* by Theo Colborn, a study was recorded of the effects of a pesticide spill that occurred in 1980 in Lake Apopka, which is near my home.[2] I've driven by this lake many times.

Following the spill, the alligator population in Lake Apopka was studied by biologists from the University of Florida, along with biologists from the U.S. Fish and Wildlife Service and the Florida Game and Freshwater Fish Commission. They found that the female alligators' ovaries had abnormalities in both their eggs and their egg follicles, similar to what happens in humans who are exposed to DES early in childhood.[3]

There were structural abnormalities in the male alligators as well. Their testes and penises were smaller than normal. In addition, the males also had elevated levels of estrogen and significantly reduced levels of testosterone.[4]

The pesticide spill also affected turtles in Lake Apopka. Researchers found a striking absence of male turtles. They found many female turtles in the lake and many turtles that were neither male nor female, which resulted from a large-scale hormonal disruption due to the pesticides in the lake. The turtles that should have become males ended up being neither male nor female, and therefore remained unable to reproduce.[5]

Growth hormones and estrogens are also given to animals to fatten them up and are probably causing earlier menarche and heavier, taller children. Men today have lower sperm counts, so it is actually affecting the ability to procreate.

You can find xeno-hormones in the following:

- Alcohol
- Fingernail polish
- Fingernail polish remover
- Paints
- Varnishes
- Industrial cleaners
- Degreasers
- Glues
- Dry-cleaning fluids
- Pesticides
- Herbicides
- Plastics
- PCBs (certain toxic chemical compounds)
- Emulsifiers in cosmetics and soaps

These chemicals actually fool your body into thinking they are estrogen by binding to estrogen receptors, which can then create the symptoms of estrogen dominance.

There are other common causes of estrogen dominance as well. These include:

- Too much stress
- Hysterectomy
- Tubal ligation

- Some birth control pills
- Going through premenopause when your body continues to secrete estrogen but its level of progesterone is significantly depleted because of not ovulating
- A poorly functioning liver
- Drinking too much alcohol
- Excessive use of prescription medications
- Excessive use of over-the-counter medications such as Tylenol that can place a strain on the liver

Chronic constipation can also lead to higher estrogen levels because both xeno-estrogens and regular estrogens can be reabsorbed back into the body.

Estrogen As an Agricultural Additive

If you've ever traveled through farm country, you've probably enjoyed picture-perfect scenes of healthy fat cows and other livestock grazing in the pastures throughout this great country of ours. What you may not have been aware of is that most of these animals are much larger and fatter than nature ever intended.

Estrogen and other hormones are commonly given to livestock in order to fatten them up.

American farmers routinely use hormones including estrogen, progesterone and testosterone so that the cattle will grow faster, larger and produce more milk and more meat.

In addition, xeno-hormones, which are estrogen-like chemicals, are commonly present in the feed. These synthetic hormones become concentrated in the fatty tissues of the animals we eat. So it's not difficult to see why so many women are suffering with mood swings and PMS pain and discomfort because of hormone imbalances. It's nearly impossible to eat a hamburger or drink a glass of milk that's not tainted with synthetic estrogen that may cause estrogen dominance.

Problems With Progesterone

Often a woman stops ovulating when she's in her thirties, although she may not be aware of it. This can throw her body out of balance. When she stops ovulating, too little progesterone is then produced. Progesterone levels decline, and the hormone estrogen becomes dominant.

The progesterone in your body can be converted to cortisol, which is similar to cortisone, and it can also be converted to the male hormone testosterone. Higher levels of cortisol are produced in your body when you are under a great deal of stress. But producing cortisol depends on your body having enough progesterone. If you have stopped ovulating and your progesterone levels have decreased, then your body may not be able to produce enough cortisol. That's why over time low progesterone levels can eventually lead to chronic fatigue and exhaustion.

As it makes its way along its chemical path, progesterone can be transformed directly or indirectly into other hormones, including estrogen, testosterone, cortisol and aldosterone. Aldosterone helps your body to maintain the correct balance of minerals. A lack of cortisol will lead to low blood sugar, allergies, immune dysfunction and arthritis as well as fatigue and exhaustion. So you can see how important it is to your health as a woman to have the proper levels of these steroid hormones.

> *You will experience all these blessings if you obey the LORD your God.*
> —DEUTERONOMY 28:2

The Powerful Benefits of Progesterone

Although many women worry about getting enough estrogen during and following menopause, the decrease in progesterone in your body is actually significantly greater than the decrease in estrogen.

Progesterone aids your body by keeping estrogen levels balanced and by preventing the dangerous and uncomfortable side effects of estrogen dominance. Let's take a look at some of the powerful benefits progesterone provides.

- It helps to protect you from developing fibrocystic breast disease.
- It helps to restore your sex drive.
- It helps to prevent breast, uterine and ovarian cancer.
- It helps to balance blood sugar levels.

In addition to these mighty benefits, by balancing cortisol levels progesterone can also help to improve your energy level, your immune function, allergy resistance and also to lower blood sugar. But that's not all. Progesterone also helps to build bone, thus preventing osteoporosis. And since it is found in the neurons in the brain, adequate progesterone levels may even help you to concentrate better.

Conclusion

Did you think you understood all about your monthly cycles before you picked up this booklet? Are you surprised about how much you still have to learn? Your body is so incredibly complex that you could study it for a lifetime and still learn new information each time you did. All of us could!

God has blessed you with a healthy body that is a marvelous creation and an incredible work of divine genius. In addition, He created you in His own image, with intelligence and stewardship of the great blessings He has given to you.

You are, indeed, richly blessed by God. Proverbs 10:22 says, "The Lord's blessing is our greatest wealth" (TLB). The New American Standard version adds to that verse, "And He adds no sorrow to it."

God has not given you the blessing of your body only to add the sorrow of painful PMS. Instead, He has provided some of the wisdom and tools you will find throughout the following chapters to help you master your symptoms and rise above their discomfort.

A BIBLE CURE PRAYER
FOR YOU

Dear Lord, thank You for all Your many marvelous blessings upon my life. Help me to see and understand that I am a blessed creature in every way—that there is no part of my life that is not powerfully and wonderfully blessed. Help me to apply the tools You have provided with a grateful heart. In Jesus' name, amen.

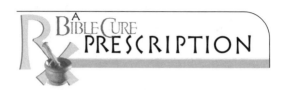

Personalize your own "version" of blessings from God by filling your name in the blanks.

> And all these blessings shall overtake _____, if she will obey the LORD her God. _____ is blessed in the city and blessed in the country. _____ is blessed in the offspring of her body and the produce of her ground and the offspring of her beasts, the increase of her herd and the young of your flock [in her wealth]. _____ is blessed in her basket and kneading bowl [in her food]. _____ is blessed when she comes in, and blessed when she goes out. [Everywhere she goes she is blessed.]
>
> The LORD will cause _____'s enemies who rise up against her to be defeated [even physical enemies such as PMS]; they shall come out against _____ one way and shall flee before her seven ways. The LORD will

command the blessing upon
_____ in her barns and in all that
she puts her hand to, and He will bless
her in the land which the LORD her God
gives her [her inheritance, which
include physical and spiritual things]
. . . And the LORD will make _____
abound in prosperity, in the offspring of
_____'s body and in the offspring
of her beast and in the produce of her
ground [in all of her possessions].

—TAKEN FROM
DEUTERONOMY 28:2–8, 11, ____
(WRITE YOUR INITIALS FOR BIBLE VERSION)

Put this on your refrigerator and on your bath-
room mirror. Read it aloud to yourself every day
for one month.

Chapter 2

The Truth
About Nutrition

S ome folks really believe that God wants them to struggle, to starve and to have the last place and the smallest portion possible. But this kind of mentality about God is simply a lie. The truth is absolutely the opposite. God richly blesses us in a wonderfully extravagant way with everything good in heaven and earth—including the food we eat! The Bible says, "But I would feed you with the best of foods. I would satisfy you with wild honey from the rock" (Ps. 81:16).

God doesn't intend for you to live your life eating bland, undesirable food. He has created the earth with a banquet of tempting and delicious choices not only to satisfy your taste buds, but also to support your health in every way as well.

Let's look at some satisfying choices that you can make in your diet that will help your body to triumph over the symptoms of PMS.

A Garden of Eden of Delightful Choices

The Garden of Eden was a place where Adam and Eve feasted on a banquet of natural delights prepared by their loving Creator. They were truly and wonderfully blessed. Everything they ate in that exotic place was not only genuinely delicious, but it was also completely nourishing to their bodies.

Think about Adam and Eve and the Garden of Eden as you consider reestablishing your eating habits to help your body to regain the natural balance that was created by God for you to enjoy.

You can reduce your body's estrogen levels by eating the following whole, fresh natural foods:

- Fruits
- Vegetables
- Whole grains
- Legumes (beans)
- Nuts and seeds

Stay Close to the Garden of Eden

Stay close to the Garden of Eden when you make your selections. In other words, the more processed and man-made an item is, the more likely it is to throw your body out of kilter hormonally. In practical terms, that means you should limit the following:

- Sugar
- Refined, processed carbohydrates such as white bread
- Instant potatoes
- White rice
- Hydrogenated, saturated and excessive amounts of polyunsaturated fats

This doesn't mean that you have to deprive yourself of an occasional sweet treat. Just try to be sure that most of your diet choices are close to the garden, which means they are whole, fresh, unprocessed and completely natural. By carefully limiting the above foods, you should be able to balance your estrogen level as well as your cortisol level, thus relieving your PMS symptoms.

Sober Truth About Sugar

Women who eat more sugar tend to experience more symptoms of PMS.

If you eat high-sugar foods and processed carbohydrates, your blood sugar will rise along with a corresponding rise in insulin. But when insulin rises, it causes your blood sugar to plummet even lower than it was when you first started eating. Now a release of adrenaline and cortisol is triggered that will tend to cause an imbalance of progesterone, thus leading to symptoms of PMS.

You can see what a vicious cycle this is. The insulin your body releases to bring down sugar will actually make you think you are craving more sugar. When you eat more sugar or highly processed carbohydrates, the cycle starts all over again. One of the many losers in this trap is your hormonal balance, because each time your sugar rises and drops, your hormones are also directly affected.

That's why it is critically important that you drastically limit all sugars and highly processed carbohydrates such as white bread, rice cakes, cereals and other high-glycemic foods. Choose foods that are low on the glycemic index. For a complete glycemic listing of foods, refer to *The Bible Cure for Weight Loss and Muscle Gain.*

Generation J (for Junk Food)

We are a junk food generation. But I wonder what would have happened if Adam and Eve had been given junk food. Would they have eaten it? Would they have liked it? I certainly doubt it. As a matter of fact, when you get accustomed to giving your body plenty of whole, natural foods, you may begin to look at junk foods as not being real food at all!

Therefore, the Garden of Eden principle really applies to junk food. To live above the miserable symptoms of PMS, drastically cut down on the amount of junk food you eat.

Junk foods are high in sugar and refined, processed carbohydrates, which stimulate insulin release. This leads to the release of adrenaline and cortisol, which causes an imbalance in progesterone.

> *Your throne is founded on two strong pillars— righteousness and justice. Unfailing love and truth walk before you as attendants.*
> —PSALM 89:14

As cortisol levels rise, they will eventually cause a decrease in progesterone levels.

The Facts About Fats

Twinkies, lunch pies and cookies tend to be made from hydrogenated fats such as margarine. In addition, other junk foods such as French fries and potato chips are made from polyunsaturated fats such as sunflower oil, safflower oil and corn oil. These fats lead to elevated amounts of inflammatory prostaglandins—potent hormones that trigger inflammation and raise cortisol levels.

Just as hydrogenated fats are the most harmful fats (these are found in margarine, cakes, pies, cookies and chips), there are also good fats that help to improve symptoms of PMS. These are:

- Black currant oil
- Borage oil
- Evening primrose oil

These oils contain high amounts of GLA. GLA is a very important fatty acid that stimulates the production of the good prostaglandins. They actually decrease inflammation, leading to a decrease in cortisol.

Extra-virgin olive oil is excellent for stir-frying and as a salad dressing. Good fats are also found in seeds and nuts, flaxseed oil, fish oils and fatty fish such as salmon, mackerel, herring, halibut and tuna. However, nuts go rancid easily; they should be kept in an airtight container and stored in a refrigerator or freezer.

To begin your new, closer-to-the-Garden of Eden nutritional lifestyle, limit bad fats and add good ones.

Straight Talk
About Saturated Fats

Fatty meats and whole-milk products contain xeno-estrogens, which can load your body up with even more estrogen and create huge hormonal imbalances that may result in severe PMS.

Avoid saturated fats, which are fatty meats and dairy products such as butter, cheese and whole milk.

Choose organic, fat-free varieties of milk, butter and cheese, and choose organic eggs. Read the labels carefully. Many of these varieties have been produced free of hormones, but not all. In addition, free-range meats that have been raised to be free of synthetic hormones can also be purchased. Many grocery store are now stocking these varieties. If you can't find them at your local grocery store, look for them at your favorite health food store, but always choose the leanest cuts.

Xeno-Estrogens and Fats

Animal fats are our main source of oral intake of xeno-estrogens. These are especially high in fatty beef, whole milk, butter, cheese, pork and other very fatty cuts of meat. Since xeno-estrogens accumulate in the fatty tissues, when we consume fatty pieces of meat or whole-milk products, we are not only consuming saturated fat, but also xeno-estrogens.

Because of our continued exposure, xeno-estrogens are slowly collecting in our tissues, especially the fatty tissues. This is probably the main reason we are witnessing such a major epidemic of premenopause in younger women and breast cancer in middle-aged and older women.

Here are some tips to help rid your body of xeno-estrogens:

- Choose lean, free-range meats since the fat in regular meat is usually high in xeno-estrogens.
- Choose organic foods because they are normally free of hormones and pesticides.
- Choose fat-free or low-fat dairy products.

A Bible Cure RECIPE

DR. COLBERT'S PMS-BUSTING SOY SHAKE

Here's a delicious shake that you can make every morning. Not only will it help you to get your body in better balance, but it will help you to start your day in a healthy way, too!

1 scoop soy protein with isoflavones
½–1 frozen banana
1 cup soy milk or water

1 Tbsp. granular lecithin

2–3 tsp. finely ground flaxseeds (grind the flaxseeds in a coffee grinder)

Blend together for 2–3 minutes at high speed. For additional sweetening, you may add a couple of drops of Stevia as needed. Enjoy!

Speaking Sincerely About Soy

Although you want to shun foods that are packed with synthetic estrogens, there are estrogenic foods that will actually greatly help you. These are called phytoestrogens. Phytoestrogens are found in some plants, and eating them can really help to get you hormonally balanced.

Plant estrogens bind to estrogen receptors, but these plant estrogens are only about one-hundredth as strong as estrogen. Although you might

> *Work hard so God can approve you. Be a good worker, one who does not need to be ashamed and who correctly explains the word of truth.*
> —2 Timothy 2:15

think that eating plant estrogens might increase the amount of estrogen in your body, the effect is usually the opposite. Since many women with premenopause and PMS also have estrogen dominance, here's what happens. Your body receives the milder phytoestrogen, which binds to the estrogen receptor and tends to reduce your high estrogen level. That's why Oriental women who eat diets with a lot of phytoestrogens experience very little PMS. On the other hand, if your estrogen level is too low, the phytoestrogens will also bind to the estrogen receptors, causing an increase in estrogenic effect. So you see that these marvelous foods work hard to help your body balance your hormones.

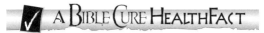

✓ A BIBLE CURE HEALTHFACT

Japanese women have few difficulties and symptoms of menopause. Hot flashes and night sweats are significantly lower than among Western women. In a cross-cultural sample with over eight thousand Massachusetts women and thirteen hundred Canadian women, twelve hundred Japanese women ages forty-five to fifty-five were compared. Writing in *Psychosomatic Medicine,* medical anthropologist Margaret Lock, Ph.D., reported that these Japanese women have sociological and biological factors such as diet that lower the symptoms of menopause. Some researchers have suggested that the Asian diet with higher quantities of phytoestrogens lessens the symptoms of menopause.[1]

The best known source for phytoestrogens is soy. You can eat soy products such as miso, tempeh, tofu, soy milk, soy protein, soy nuts or soy sprouts, or you may take a supplement containing approximately 50 milligrams of iso-flavones per day. The isoflavone genistine is the primary phytoestrogen in soy. Just be careful that you're not allergic to soy products—some folks are allergic to them and must avoid them.

A BIBLE CURE HEALTH TIP

The Sources of Soy

Don't know tofu from tempeh? Here are some of the most common soy foods, along with a few suggestions for using them.

Meat substitutes—If you want to cut back on meat while getting more soy, look for "mock" meats prepared in the form of cold cuts, bacon, sausage, franks and burgers. These are mainly made from soy, and in some cases they are virtually indistinguishable from the real thing.

Soy flour—Made from roasted, ground soybeans, soy flour can be used to replace some of the wheat flour used for baking. Nutritionists advise buying defatted soy flour, which contains less fat and more protein than the full-fat variety.

Soy milk—A creamy, milklike drink made from ground, soaked soybeans and water, it's sold plain and in a variety of flavors. Some people prefer "lite" soy milk. It's lower in fat than the regular kind, but it may contain fewer of the protective phyto-estrogens.

Tempeh—These chunky, tender cakes are made from fermented soybeans that have been laced with mold, giving them their distinctive smoky, nutty flavor. You can grill tempeh or add it to spaghetti sauce, chili or casseroles.

Texturized soy protein—Made from soy flour, this meat substitute can replace part or all of the meat in meatloaf, burgers and chili.

Tofu—A creamy white, soft, cheeselike food made from curdled soy milk, tofu can be used in virtually anything from soups to desserts. You will find soft and firm varieties of tofu at most supermarkets in the produce section.

Other soy foods are available at specialty and health food stores.[2]

Correcting
Misunderstandings About Caffeine

For years we heard that caffeine was OK, and then they told us it wasn't. Now some are saying caffeine is OK in moderation. So much has been said, but what's correct?

Caffeine may not be a problem for many individuals, but if your body is laboring under the weight of hormonal imbalance, you would be much better off to drastically limit your caffeine intake.

If you have PMS or are premenopausal, either avoid or significantly decrease your consumption of caffeinated beverages. Caffeine is associated with fibrocystic breast disease and breast tenderness. Drinking too much coffee and other caffeinated drinks can also result in irritability, insomnia, anxiety and depression.

Frank Talk About Fiber

Making sure that your diet has enough fiber is also very important for controlling PMS and premenopause symptoms. Fiber helps to eliminate excess estrogen through the colon. High-fiber foods also help to lower the glycemic index and thus help to break you out of that awful cycle of eating sugar and craving starches.

Foods high in fiber include:

- Beans
- Peas
- Fruits
- Legumes
- Lentils
- Whole grains

Speaking Out About Salt

Finally, lowering your salt intake is vital. Since many PMS and premenopause symptoms are related to water retention, watching your salt intake can really make a difference.

Eating too much salt increases water retention, abdominal bloating and edema. These common symptoms of premenopause and PMS are often caused by elevated cortisol and aldosterone levels. By decreasing your salt intake, most of these symptoms can be completely relieved.

Lower your salt by limiting high-sodium foods, which are mainly processed foods, and by eating more fresh fruits and

> *May you be blessed by the LORD, who made heaven and earth.*
> —PSALM 115:15

vegetables. Oh, and one more thing . . . keep the salt shaker off the table!

In Conclusion

God cares about what you eat, and He cares about the way you eat. That's why as your divine Creator He filled the earth with wonderfully delicious natural foods and other things to keep you healthy and satisfied. You may not live in the Garden of Eden, but many of the same nutritional choices that were provided there are still available to you. The Garden of Eden was a place of beauty and balance, and as you consider your

Creator and the truth about His love and care for you—body, mind and spirit—your life can begin to recapture something of that wonderful place. You are truly blessed!

A BIBLE CURE PRAYER
FOR YOU

Dear God, thank You for the truth about Your blessings upon my life. Thank You that You created the earth as a garden of natural delights to strengthen, nourish and restore my body. Help me to make the dietary choices necessary to bring my body back into the perfect balance that You intended for it to have. In Jesus' name, amen.

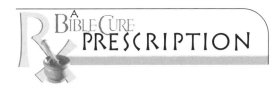

Toward a Healthy, Nutritional Lifestyle

List five types of foods you will avoid eating in order to help your body rise above PMS.

_____

_____

List at least five healthy choices of foods you will make this week as you plan your menus.

_____

_____

Write a prayer asking God to help you make right nutritional choices.

_____

_____

_____

_____

Chapter 3

The Truth About Exercise and Lifestyle

Have you ever looked around and thought that the blessings of God seem to be for everyone else except you? One person is blessed with health, another individual is blessed with beauty, while someone else is slender and athletic.

If you have believed that God has blessed others more than you, then you have believed a lie. God is not a respecter of persons. The Bible says, "I most certainly understand now that God is not one to show partiality" (Acts 10:34, NAS).

Even if you are not presently walking in them, God's blessings upon your life include glowing with a sense of health and well-being, looking vibrant and being the very best you can be! God's words of blessing for your life are absolutely true. The Bible also says, "For the word of the LORD holds true, and everything he does is worthy of our trust" (Ps. 33:4).

If the mood swings and emotional roller coaster of PMS have weighed you down and diminished your self-esteem, some lifestyle changes could be in order. With God's help, implementing a few lifestyle changes can refresh your attitude, outlook, health and even your physical appearance! Let's take a look at this exciting and sometimes even fun tool for overcoming the symptoms of PMS.

Taking Mastery

PMS can make you feel as if you are completely out of control. But with God's help, you can take back the mastery over your life and body, beginning this very minute. Your body will respond to your control as you master it. The apostle Paul understood this mind-set. Look at what he said:

> Remember that in a race everyone runs, but only one person gets the prize. You also must run in such a way that you will win. All athletes practice strict self-control. They do it to win a prize that will fade away, but we do it for an eternal prize. So I run straight to the goal with purpose in every step. I am not like a

boxer who misses his punches. I discipline my body like an athlete, training it to do what it should. Otherwise, I fear that after preaching to others I myself might be disqualified.

—1 Corinthians 9:24–27

Paul wasn't the greatest apostle by accident. He made up his mind, and God helped him to be all that he could be. God will help you, too!

Your body needs to be maintained in divine health through weight loss and exercise. Obesity is a major cause of estrogen dominance, which leads to pre-menopausal symptoms. As you recall, fatty tissue will cause an increased production of estrogen.

> *When the Spirit of truth comes, he will guide you into all truth. He will not be presenting his own ideas; he will be telling you what he has heard.*
>
> —John 16:13

Do You Love to Walk?

I recommend taking a twenty- to thirty-minute brisk walk every other day. Or try another type of fresh air exercise that you can enjoy at least three to four times a week. Why not purchase yourself a bicycle?

Regular exercise can make all the difference in the world when you're battling hormonal imbalance and PMS symptoms. It helps to keep your metabolism high, which prevents weight gain, and it melts away stress.

A Walking Program

Here's a walking program to help get you exercising. Don't look at walking as work. Instead, choose to see it as "your time," a special time for you to get away and enjoy the outdoors, fresh air and the wonders of God's creation.

Always get a medical checkup before starting an exercise program. Begin walking at a pace that is comfortable for you. However, you should walk briskly enough so that you cannot sing, but not so briskly that you cannot talk.

A BIBLE CURE HEALTH TIP

A Simple Walking Program

(NOTE: Each column indicates the number of minutes to walk. Complete three exercise sessions each week. If you find a particular week's pattern tiring, repeat it before going on to the next pattern. You do not have to complete the walking program in twelve weeks.)

Week	—Walk	—Walk Briskly	—Walk	—Minutes
1	5	5	5	15
2	5	7	5	17
3	5	9	5	19
4	5	11	5	21
5	5	13	5	23
6	5	15	5	25
7	5	18	5	28
8	5	20	5	30
9	5	23	5	33
10	5	26	5	36
11	5	28	5	38
12	5	30	5	40

Week 13 and thereafter: Check your pulse periodically to see if you are exercising within your target zone. As you get more in shape, try exercising within the upper range of your target zone. Gradually increase your brisk walking time from 30 to 60 minutes, three or four times a week. Remember that your goal is to get the benefits you are seeking and enjoy your activity.

You can also obtain a heart rate monitor that straps around your chest to calculate your heart rate while you walk. The following Health Tip shows you how to calculate your target heart zone.

Your Predicted Heart Rate

Calculate your predicted heart rate using this formula:

220 minus [your age] = _____

x .65 = _____ x .80 = _____

Calculate your target heart zone using this formula:

220 minus [your age] = _____

x .65 = _____

[This is your minimum.]

220 minus [your age] = _____

x .80 = _____

[This is your maximum.]

This example may help: To calculate the target heart zone for a 40-year-old man, subtract the age (40) from 220 (220- 40=180). Multiply 180 by .65, which equals 117. Then multiply 180 by .80, which equals 144. A 40-year-old man's target heart rate zone is 117–144 beats per minute.

Staying With It

You may be thinking, *I've tried many exercise programs, but I never hang in there long enough to get results. I always quit too soon.* Here's a tip: Make your walking program a vital part of your day. Too many people get into trouble when they save exercising for their spare time. If you wait until you get around to it, you probably never will. Schedule exercise during the day as you would schedule an appointment—and do not break that appointment. Choose an exercise activity that you truly enjoy.

Recharge your body every night by getting at least seven to eight hours of good, restful sleep. This will recharge not only your body, but also your mind. It will help to prevent irritability, anxiety, depression and fatigue.

Learning to Deal With Stress

If you have PMS, you're probably dealing with a lot of stress. Most women with PMS are almost always under too much stress.

Excessive stress raises levels of the hormones cortisol and adrenaline, which leads to decreased levels of progesterone and symptoms of PMS, and it will also raise the levels of aldosterone. Aldosterone regulates the minerals in the cells. Too much stress causes the adrenal glands to secrete excessive amounts of aldosterone, which may raise your blood pressure by triggering the kidneys to retain sodium and to excrete potassium and magnesium. This may also lead to water retention, bloating in the abdomen and edema (or swelling) in the lower extremities.

As you can see, many of the symptoms of PMS are caused by elevated levels of the hormones cortisol, adrenaline and aldosterone, all of which are triggered by too much stress. Stress also raises the levels of another hormone called prolactin. Prolactin stimulates the breasts to make milk, but it also lowers the production of progesterone.

Therefore, lowering levels of the hormones cortisol, adrenaline, aldosterone and prolactin by controlling stress or learning to live with stress is critically important in managing symptoms of PMS. We have seen how stress can cause an imbalance of the hormones in the body. Therefore, in order to balance hormones you must get a handle on your stress.

Stress Busters

Regular exercise will go a long way in reducing your stress and helping your body to reclaim its proper hormonal balance. Another stress buster, and perhaps the most important, is adequate restful sleep (at least eight hours a night), along with adequate rest and relaxation. Learn to relax and practice it regularly. Learn to set limits and say "no" to decrease your number of commitments. Honor the Sabbath by taking at least one day off a week to rest and rejuvenate your body.

Here are some other stress-busting ideas that you may not have considered.

Take a steamy hot aromatherapy bath.

Here's a great idea to melt away stress after a grueling day at work or carpooling. At the end of a particularly stressful day, take a candlelight aromatherapy bath. Fill the tub with steamy hot water and fragrant aromatherapy oil such as lavender. Play some soft, instrumental music and relax as your stress melts away.

Aromatherapy, or the fragrant use of essential oils, is an easy and soothing way to treat a number of PMS symptoms. Smell has a powerful influence on the body and mind, possibly because the olfactory nerve is in direct contact with the emotional center of the brain. So it's not surprising that many women report that aromatherapy relieves the pain, anxiety and depression they experience with PMS.

> *For the law was given through Moses; God's unfailing love and faithfulness came through Jesus Christ.*
> —JOHN 1:17

Melt Away Stress
With the Scent of Lavender

Essential oils can be added directly to your bath water. Here's how:

- Add 5–10 drops of essential oils to hot water while filling your bath.

- Do not combine essential oils with other bath oils or soap.

- Make sure to soak in the tub for at least 20 minutes to get the aromatic benefits.

You can find essential oils at health food stores. The following essential oils have properties that are especially beneficial in relieving PMS symptoms.

Lavender. At first this oil may pep you up a little. But as you soak for a few minutes, you'll find that it calms you. It relieves nervous tension, depression and insomnia.

Geranium. Combine a couple drops of this with lavender. It has a calming effect.

Rosemary. This one helps circulation. Use it alone or with lavender to relieve depression.

Have a cup of herbal tea.

Sometimes all it takes to calm your nerves and get you through a particularly stressful moment is making a hot cup of herbal tea. There are many different varieties for you to choose from, and many are absolutely delicious. Just remember to sweeten your tea with Stevia instead of sugar or honey, and relax and enjoy!

Here are some herbal teas you may try:

- **Chasteberry.** The recorded use of chasteberry for PMS dates back to the time of Hippocrates.

- **Skullcap.** This tea is well known as a sedative and remedy for PMS.

- **Dong quai.** In Chinese lore, this tea was known as the female tonic and is very effective in reducing tension and relieving cramps.[1]

These herbs can be purchased at a health food store and stored in a tightly sealed container. Use 1 to 2 teaspoons of the herb for each 8-ounce cup of hot, but not boiling, water. Cover and let steep for ten to fifteen minutes. You may have this tea twice a day.

You can also find specially prepared PMS teas at health food and grocery stores.

Light Up Your Life

Many women with PMS have depressive symptoms similar to those experienced by people with SAD (seasonal affective disorder). This condition starts most often in the winter or fall. But the interesting key to this disorder is sunlight. When a person with SAD increases her amount of exposure to sunlight, SAD symptoms simply vanish.

Interestingly, PMS works similarly for some individuals. So get out of doors more often. If you work in an office with no windows and leave for work in the dark and drive back home in the dark, well, that can simply be depressing. Why not try taking your lunch hours in a park or pack a lunch and pull your car up to a lake and listen to music and read a book? Getting a few moments away from the stress and in the sunlight might do wonders for your stress![2]

Reduce Your Xeno-Estrogens

Since your level of stress is also linked to your exposure to xeno-estrogens, I strongly recommend that you stop using pesticides in your home.

Here are some other ways you can reduce your exposure to xeno-estrogens. Avoid or at least decrease your exposure to:

- All solvents including alcohol
- Fingernail polish
- Industrial cleaners
- Degreasers
- Paints and mineral spirits
- Some air fresheners

In addition, don't drink hot beverages or eat hot soups from plastic cups or bowls. Don't microwave your

> *Teach me your ways, O Lord, that I may live according to your truth!*
> —Psalm 86:11

food in plastic containers since this will also release xeno-estrogens. For cleaners, choose natural products instead of petrochemical products. For information on this subject, read my book *What You Don't Know May Be Killing You.*

In Conclusion

Even if your life is hectic and stressful, your body does not have to be dramatically impacted by it. These lifestyle tips are only a few of the many ways you can learn to live and cope with stress—even a lot of stress—without being stressed out.

Learn to see the busy pace of your life as a blessing of fruitfulness given to you by God. In addition, more important than any of these lifestyle tips is learning to go to God for help. He will always hear you and He will not forsake you. When stress starts to get the better of you, call out to Him in prayer. You won't be disappointed.

A BIBLE CURE PRAYER
FOR YOU

Lord, You are my shepherd; I have every-thing I need.

Thank You for letting me rest in green meadows and leading me beside peaceful streams.

I praise You for renewing my strength. Lord, guide me along right paths, that I might bring honor to Your name.

Even when I walk through the dark valley of death, I will not be afraid, for You are close beside me. Your rod and Your staff protect and comfort me.

You prepare a feast for me in the presence of my enemies. You welcome me as a guest, anointing my head with oil. My cup overflows with blessings.

Surely Your goodness and unfailing love will pursue me all the days of my life, and I will live in the house of the Lord forever. Amen.

—ADAPTED FROM PSALM 23

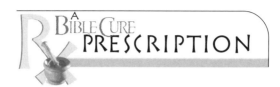

In order to rest properly, you must eliminate certain things from your life. Check those things below that you will eliminate and avoid:

- ❏ Caffeine
- ❏ Sleeping pills
- ❏ Alcohol

Check the positive steps you will take:

- ❏ Set limits and decrease your number of commitments.
- ❏ Get seven to eight hours of sleep regularly.
- ❏ Rest while taking a bath with lavender oil and soothing music.

Write a prayer thanking God for His rest, care and peace in your life:

_____

_____

_____

Chapter 4

The Truth About Supplements

If you have believed that God has provided nothing for you to relieve your PMS, mood swings, depression, cramping and monthly discomfort, then you have believed a lie. With supernatural genius, God wisely created the earth and filled it with everything you need.

> And God said, "Look! I have given you the seed-bearing plants throughout the earth and all the fruit trees for your food. And I have given all the grasses and other green plants to the animals and birds for their food." And so it was. Then God looked over all he had made, and he saw that it was excellent in every way.
> —GENESIS 1:29–31

You too are God's unique creation, and your

56

body is a masterful balance of artistry and chemistry. You were intricately and wonderfully made by Him! The Bible states, "You made all the delicate, inner parts of my body and knit me together in my mother's womb. Thank you for making me so wonderfully complex! Your workmanship is marvelous—and how well I know it. You watched me as I was being formed in utter seclusion, as I was woven together in the dark of the womb" (Ps. 139:13–15).

The divine Creator also richly supplied countless vitamins and minerals that are uniquely programmed by God to help your body function at peak performance—including helping it maintain a delicate hormonal balance. Although vitamins and minerals are found in some measure in the foods we eat, taking supplemental vitamins and minerals will both strengthen your body and restore it back into balance.

> *Truth springs up from the earth, and righteousness smiles down from heaven.*
> —PSALM 85:11

The Vitamin and Mineral Maze

Vitamins and minerals are important for bringing your body back into the right hormonal balance.

But if you're like many of us, looking at health food and grocery store shelves lined with bottles of vitamins and other supplements can leave you feeling a little mystified. Here is some practical and easy information about some of these powerful natural substances that can have you feeling better in no time.

A comprehensive multivitamin/ multimineral supplement

Improve your PMS and premenopause symptoms with zinc, vitamin B_6, all the other B-complex vitamins and 400 milligrams per day of magnesium. All of these can be found in a good comprehensive multivitamin/multimineral supplement such as Divine Health Multivitamins. These nutrients help to balance the hormones in the body.

Take a good comprehensive supplement daily.

Natural progesterone cream

Natural progesterone cream can help balance your hormones and reduce PMS symptoms. It also helps to reduce the pain of tender, swollen breasts. In addition, most premenopausal women are very often estrogen dominant. Those high estrogen levels can cause you to crave carbohydrates and sugars and make you gain weight. You can balance the estrogen levels by supplementing with natural progesterone cream.

Use 3 percent progesterone cream. Apply ¼ teaspoon once or twice a day, especially from days twelve through twenty-six in the menstrual cycle. Day one is the first day of the menstrual period. For tender, swollen breasts rub the cream directly on breasts.

Vitamin E

Vitamin E can help to reduce breast tenderness. If this is an ongoing severe problem, you may also need to have your dosage of birth control medication decreased or eliminated.

Take 400–800 IUs daily to help decrease breast tenderness. Purchase natural vitamin E, which is called d-alpha-tocopherol.

Chasteberry

For irregular periods the herb chasteberry, which is also called vitex, can help. This herb actually helps to stimulate the hypothalamus to increase the hormone LH. This, in turn, may help to stimulate the production of progesterone.

Take 200 to 225 milligrams of a standardized extract of vitex a day or drink chasteberry tea.

GLA

GLA is found in evening primrose oil, borage oil and black currant oil. GLA may be helpful in controlling cyclic breast tenderness. The body needs adequate amounts of B_6, magnesium and zinc in order to make enough of its own GLA.

The usual dose of GLA is 200–400 milligrams a day. Or you may take 4 grams of evening primrose oil a day or about 2 grams of borage oil a day. Be patient, however, for it may take a few months to notice the benefits of this.

Help for Excessive Bleeding

If your PMS is accompanied by heavy bleeding, get a pelvic ultrasound to rule out large uterine fibroids. These are commonly associated with heavy bleeding.

To help control heavy bleeding you will need a stronger natural progesterone cream such as 6 or 10 percent.

- Use ¼ teaspoon of 6 or 10 percent progesterone cream twice a day on days twelve through twenty-six to better control heavy bleeding.

- 500–1000 milligrams of Vitamin C with

bioflavonoids, three times a day, may help decrease blood loss from heavy menstruation.

- If heavy bleeding continues, have a complete blood count taken together with a serum iron and ferritin level blood test to see if you need an iron supplement. You may need to supplement with iron to prevent or to treat iron-deficiency anemia.

Loss of Sex Drive

Estrogen dominance will not only cause you to gain weight, but it will often cause a loss of sex drive. As excess estrogen may suppress sex drive, the hormones progesterone and testosterone will usually increase it. That's why I often place PMS sufferers who are experiencing a loss of sex drive on both natural progesterone cream and natural testosterone cream. This usually will both balance your estrogen and dramatically improve your sex drive.

Helpful Herbs for
PMS and Premenopause

Dong quai is commonly recommend for menstrual cramps, PMS and hot flashes. It may be taken in capsules, tablets, tinctures or teas. A common dose is 3 grams a day.

Black cohosh has been used for over forty years. It helps to decrease many of the symptoms of menopause, including hot flashes, depression and insomnia. The black cohosh product called Remifemin is a German product and is of very high quality.

> *The LORD's blessings be upon you; we bless you in the LORD's name.*
> —PSALM 129:8

Take one tablet twice a day.

Especially
for Premenopause

If you are struggling with premenopause, your approach to hormonal balance may vary slightly from the advice for PMS given above. Add the following to the above prescription.

Estrogen

If your estrogen levels are low, or if you are having symptoms including hot flashes or vaginal dryness, you should supplement with natural estrogen cream. I recommend using BiEst, which is 90 percent estriol and 10 percent estradiol.

This cream must be prescribed by a physician and must be filled at a compounding pharmacy.

For someone in your area who prescribes natural hormones, call 1-800-LEADOUT.

Pregnenolone

Pregnenolone has been called the grandmother of all steroid hormones, and it is the raw material for making progesterone.

Pregnenolone is usually taken in a dose of 30–100 milligrams a day.

Testosterone

As estrogen and progesterone decline with age, so does testosterone. This often leads to decreased sex drive. However, by supplementing with a low dose of natural testosterone cream, once or twice a day, often sex drive can be completely restored.

You must obtain this by prescription from a compounding pharmacy.

Stress-Busting Solutions

Stress plays a major role in the symptoms of PMS and premenopause. Many if not most of the symptoms of premenopause are related to stressed adrenal glands. Many women's lives are so busy with work, home, children, husband and church and social activities that they end up having too little time left to take care of themselves.

If this sounds like you, your busy, stressed-out lifestyle can cause your body's levels of epinephrine and cortisol to become elevated. Higher levels of cortisol will actually lead to decreased levels of progesterone. Elevated cortisol levels can result in weight gain, memory loss, blood sugar changes, insomnia, irritability and depression. Eventually, your adrenal glands can get so worn out that you may develop chronic fatigue, low blood pressure, allergies, low metabolic rate with cold hands and cold feet, depression, irregular periods and constant recurring infections. Remember that no supplement is as important as adequate sleep, rest and relaxation.

You may want to consider adding some stress-busting supplements to your list. Here are a few.

DSF

I also recommend an adrenal formula called DSF. This contains many vitamins and glandulars that support adrenal function. Chew one-half to one tablet twice a day. This supplement is commonly recommended by nutritional doctors and nutritionists.

DHEA

I normally place women on either DHEA, 10–25 milligrams once or twice a day, or pregnenolone, 30–100 milligrams a day.

Vitamin C

Take vitamin C, 1000 milligrams, once or twice a day.

Phosphatidyl serine

Phosphatidyl serine is very effective in lowering cortisol levels. Take 100 milligrams, one to three times a day.

If you are pregnant, or plan on becoming pregnant, stop *all* supplements and consult your physician.

Conclusion

Your body is uniquely created by divine hands and supernatural wisdom to be a blessing to you and to others around you. Your body is extremely important in God's eyes—in fact, the Bible says it is the temple of God's Spirit. First Corinthians 3:16 says:

> Don't you realize that all of you together
> are the temple of God and that the Spirit
> of God lives in you?

It's important to God that the living temple He created work at optimum performance. In addition, He loves you more than you could ever know, and He wants you to feel wonderful in body, soul and spirit. Take the time necessary to get adequate sleep and rest, take the vitamins and other supplements you need, take the time to get your body back in balance and take the time to learn more about your loving heavenly Father. You'll never regret it if you do!

A BIBLE CURE PRAYER
FOR YOU

Dear God, thank You for richly providing all the substances my body needs to get back into balance naturally. Thank You for loving me in a way that's even beyond my ability to understand. Help me to be faithful to this plan of supplements and to use them wisely. Help me to feel truly great again, all the time, so that I can serve You better. Amen.

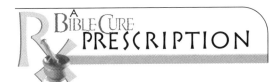

A BIBLE CURE PRESCRIPTION

Check the following vitamins and other supplements that you (along with the advice of your nutritional doctor) have determined that you need.

❑ Multivitamin/multimineral daily

❑ Natural progesterone cream (¼ tsp. 3 percent cream, once or twice daily)

❑ Vitamin E (400–800 IUs daily)

❑ Chasteberry (200–225 mg. daily)

❑ GLA (200–400 mg. a day)

❑ Dong quai (3 grams a day)

❑ Black cohosh (1 tablet, twice daily)

❑ DSF (½ to 1 tablet, twice daily)

❑ DHEA (10–25 mg. once or twice daily)

❑ Vitamin C (1000 mg. once or twice daily)

❑ Phosphatidyl serine (100 mg. one to three times a day)

❑ Pregnenolone (30–100 mg. a day)

Chapter 5

The Power of
Truth in Faith

Have you ever wondered, *What is my purpose in life?* We all have. Have you ever considered that one of the reasons God put you on this earth was simply to bless you? It's true! Remember how we noted earlier that the blessing of Abraham has come upon the Gentiles? Well, part of that blessing says, "And I will bless you, and make your name great; and so you shall be a blessing; and I will bless those who bless you, and the one who curses you I will curse" (Gen. 12:2–3, NAS). So you see, one of God's purposes in your life is simply to bless you!

Not only has God chosen to bless you, but He has also made every possible blessing in heaven available to you! The Bible says, "Praise God, the Father of our Lord Jesus Christ. In Christ, God has given us every spiritual blessing in the heavenly world" (Eph. 1:1–3, NCV).

Two of the greatest blessings of your life are God's devotion to you and His protection. "For the eyes of the LORD are on the righteous, and His ears are open to their prayers" (1 Pet. 3:12, NKJV).

Another great blessing of God upon your life is His wonderful promise of peace. God will keep you in peace through the power of faith. The Bible says, "You will keep in perfect peace all who trust in you, whose thoughts are fixed on you!" (Isa. 26:3).

You can live in all of God's wonderful blessings as an everyday fact of life through faith—

> *All these blessings shall come upon you and overtake you.*
> —DEUTERONOMY 28:2, NKJV

and you can strengthen your faith through the Word of God. "So then faith comes by hearing, and hearing by the word of God" (Rom. 10:17, NKJV). Reading the Bible, meditating upon the many scripture verses throughout this booklet and praying often will strengthen your faith and give you power to transcend every difficulty in your life—including PMS and premenopause!

Overcoming Stress
With Faith

Learn to find a place of rest in God.

When we look to God, He promises us rest. Finding a place of rest in God for your mind, spirit and body is extremely important for overcoming your symptoms of PMS.

Look at what the Bible says about God's promise of rest for you:

> The LORD is my shepherd; I have everything I need. He lets me rest in green meadows; he leads me beside peaceful streams. He renews my strength. He guides me along right paths, bringing honor to his name.
>
> —PSALM 23:1–3

Learning how to walk in God's rest is vitally important to you spiritually, mentally and physically, too.

When your body is experiencing these symptoms of adrenal exhaustion, getting a good night's rest is critically important. However, your body can feel so revved up that you are unable to sleep well. By meditating on the Word of God before you go to bed, and by quoting scriptures and singing praise and worship songs throughout your day, you will begin to renew your strength.

It is also critically important to learn how to relax. Learn how to place minimal stress on your body and mind by giving up activities that sap your strength. A good night's sleep and resting by honoring the Sabbath are critically important to restoring adrenal function.

Celebrate your life with a merry heart.

Your life is a celebration—not a struggle! But too often PMS symptoms can make you feel as if you are just barely getting by. Learn to have a merry heart—it will turn your entire outlook around.

Having a merry heart is more powerful than any medicine to restore the adrenal glands. The best medicine for overcoming stress and depression is laughter. In fact, the Bible says that a merry heart does good like a medicine. (See Proverbs 17:22.)

Norman Cousins wrote the book *Anatomy of an Illness As Perceived by the Patient* in 1979.[1] Cousins used laughter to fight a serious disease and actually laughed his way back to health. He watched funny movies such as the Marx Brothers films. He watched funny TV shows such as *Candid Camera* and read funny books.

A good belly laugh is able to stimulate all the major organs like a massage. Laughter also helps to raise your energy level and helps to pull you out of the pit of depression. Take at least a ten- to twenty-minute laughter break a day. Watch funny movies and funny TV shows. Read jokes in the newspaper, in books or magazines, and share these clean jokes with others because laughter is contagious. Instead of looking critically at a situation, find out what's funny about it.

Joy gives you strength. The Bible says, "Don't be dejected and sad, for the joy of the LORD is your strength!" (Neh. 8:10).

> *The blessing of the LORD makes a person rich, and he adds no sorrow with it.*
> —PROVERBS 10:22

You may be thinking, *That's easy for him to say. He doesn't know my circumstances!* No one but God truly knows another's circumstances, thoughts and feelings. But that doesn't matter—it's truly possible to find joy, not in circumstances, but in Christ. The Bible promises, "Thou wilt make known to me the path of life; in Thy presence is fulness of joy; in Thy right hand there are pleasures forever" (Ps. 16:11, NAS).

I encourage you to find joy in life by knowing Christ.

The average man and woman laughs about four to eight times a day. The average child laughs about 150 times a day. Strengthen your immune system by becoming more childlike and laughing more often.

Live in the power of Christ's forgiveness.

It is critically important to forgive anyone who has wronged you. Ask the Holy Spirit to bring to your remembrance any unforgiveness that is hiding in your heart.

Don't hold grudges, for they will eat away at your soul like a cancer. Take a look at what the Bible says.

> Christ did not sin or ever tell a lie. Although he was abused, he never tried to get even. And when he suffered, he made no threats. Instead, he had faith in God, who judges fairly. Christ carried the burden of our sins. He was nailed to the cross, so that we would stop sinning and start living right. By his cuts and bruises you are healed.
>
> —1 PETER 2:22–24, CEV

If you feel that you've been wronged in ways that you simply cannot forgive, consider that

Christ was completely pure and sinless and died a horrible death. Since He was punished for sin but didn't commit any, He was able to take your sin and everyone else's to the cross. He died so that you could be forgiven.

It's because of His great gift that you can find the power of forgiveness. If you have harbored hidden grudges and offenses against anyone— even God—I encourage you right this moment to give them to God. He will help you to walk in His own perfect peace.

Reject worry.

Becoming anxious about your future will only serve to weaken you physically and spiritually. Worry never overcame anything. The Bible promises:

> Always be full of joy in the Lord. I say it again—rejoice! . . . Don't worry about anything; instead, pray about everything. Tell God what you need, and thank him for all he has done. If you do this, you will experience God's peace, which is far more wonderful than the human mind can understand. His peace will guard your hearts and minds as you

live in Christ Jesus.

—Philippians 4:4, 6–7

Replace worry with the confidence and peace that God's plan for you will overcome PMS.

Pray.

Prayer is a limitless resource for filling your life with God's Spirit, wisdom and strength. He will strengthen your body and give you the determination to take the natural steps you need to take in order to walk in health. Take to heart these encouraging words from the Book of Psalms:

> I love the Lord because he hears and answers my prayers. Because he bends down and listens, I will pray as long as I have breath! Death had its hands around my throat; the terrors of the grave overtook me. I saw only trouble and sorrow. Then I called on the name of the Lord: "Please, Lord, save me!" How kind the Lord is! How good he is! So merciful, this God of ours! The Lord protects those of childlike faith; I was facing death, and then he saved me. Now I can rest again, for the Lord has been so good to me. He

has saved me from death, my eyes from tears, my feet from stumbling. And so I walk in the Lord's presence as I live here on earth!

—Psalm 116:1–9

Break the power of negative words.

Often women with PMS and premenopause speak very negative words about their symptoms. You've probably heard them. They say things such as, "I've got the curse right now." "The curse is on my life."

Sadly, such individuals don't realize that by saying such things they can actually be training their subconscious mind to see themselves as cursed. Such words are powerful and can undermine the faith in a person's heart. The Bible says, "Death and life are in the power of the tongue" (Prov. 18:21, NAS).

> *For he loves us with unfailing love; the faithfulness of the Lord endures forever.*
> —Psalm 117:2

Take a moment once in a while to listen to yourself talk. You might be surprised. If you are speaking negative words over yourself, stop. Ask God to fill your mouth with genuine appreciation and gratitude for everything in your life, including the precious gift of procreation and all that comes with it.

Trust in God's Word to heal and sustain you.

Throughout this booklet are scriptures that will strengthen and encourage you. Learn them. Speak them out loud. Let His Word bring guidance and healing into your life.

> Then they cried to the LORD in their trouble, and he saved them from their distress. He sent forth his word and healed them; he rescued them from the grave. Let them give thanks to the LORD for his unfailing love and his wonderful deeds for men.
>
> —PSALM 107:19–21, NIV

A Bible Cure Prayer
FOR YOU

Heavenly Father, thank You for creating me with the purpose of blessing me. Thank You for blessing my life with so many things. Help me walk in divine health on the path You lay before me and to know You better all along the way. Lord, help me to speak and think positive words so that my life will be helpful and refreshing to others. Give me the power to stop destructive habits and attitudes. Fill me with Your joy for life, and give me energy to take the necessary steps to stay fit, both physically and spiritually, all of my days. Amen.

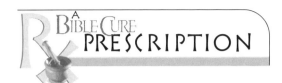

A BIBLE CURE PRESCRIPTION

What do you need to overcome in your attitude and outlook on life?

❑ Bitterness

❑ Negative thoughts

❑ Anxiety

❑ Sadness

❑ Excessive worry and stress

❑ Speaking destructive words instead of encouraging words

❑ Other: _____

Write a prayer thanking God for all the ways He has blessed your life.

_____

_____

_____

_____

_____

_____

_____

_____

Check the spiritual steps you have started in overcoming PMS:

❏ I have stopped worrying.

❏ I am praying.

❏ I am learning and applying God's Word.

❏ I am trusting God for health and strength.

❏ I am not speaking negative words.

Conclusion

You are richly and wonderfully blessed by God in many varied and precious ways. You are blessed because He loves you so much and because He sent His only Son to die for you so that you could know Him and walk in fellowship with Him.

If you feel that you don't know Him as well as you could, or if you feel that your life has become so busy that you have drifted away from the closeness to God you once had, take a moment right now and reestablish that intimacy. He is as close to you right now as the whisper of a prayer.

Remember, God has provided all you need for health and healing. He is all you need, so never stop looking to Him. Enjoy His wonderful blessings as you begin to walk in His divine health today!

—DON COLBERT, M. D.

Notes

CHAPTER 1
TRUTH THAT SETS YOU FREE

1. John Lee, *What Your Doctor May Not Tell You About Menopause* (New York: Warner Books, 1996).
2. Theo Colborn, *Our Stolen Future* (New York: Penguin Group, 1997), 150–152.
3. Ibid., 151.
4. Ibid., 151–152.
5. Ibid., 152.

CHAPTER 2
THE TRUTH ABOUT NUTRITION

1. Margaret Lock, *Psychosomatic Medicine* (July–August 1999), as cited by *Doctor's Guide* (www.pslgroup.com).
2. Selene Yeager, *New Foods for Healing* (Emmaus, PA: Rodale Press, 1998), 492.

CHAPTER 3
THE TRUTH ABOUT EXERCISE AND LIFESTYLE

1. Source obtained from the Internet: www.whole-healthmd.com.
2. Ibid.

CHAPTER 5
THE POWER OF TRUTH IN FAITH

1. Norman Cousins, *Anatomy of an Illness As Perceived by the Patient* (New York: Norton, 1979).

Don Colbert, M.D., was born in Tupelo, Mississippi. He attended Oral Roberts School of Medicine in Tulsa, Oklahoma, where he received a bachelor of science degree in biology in addition to his degree in medicine. Dr. Colbert completed his internship and residency with Florida Hospital in Orlando, Florida. He is board certified in family practice and has received extensive training in nutritional medicine.

If you would like more
information about natural and
divine healing, or information about
Divine Health Nutritional Products®,
you may contact
Dr. Colbert at:

DR. DON COLBERT

1908 Boothe Circle
Longwood, FL 32750
Telephone: 407-331-7007

Dr. Colbert's website is
www.drcolbert.com.

Pick up these other Siloam Press
books by Dr. Colbert:

Toxic Relief
Walking in Divine Health
What You Don't Know May Be Killing You

The Bible Cure® Booklet Series

The Bible Cure for ADD and Hyperactivity
The Bible Cure for Allergies
The Bible Cure for Arthritis
The Bible Cure for Cancer
The Bible Cure for Candida and Yeast Infection
The Bible Cure for Chronic Fatigue and Fibromyalgia
The Bible Cure for Depression and Anxiety
The Bible Cure for Diabetes
The Bible Cure for Headaches
The Bible Cure for Heart Disease
The Bible Cure for Heartburn and Indigestion
The Bible Cure for High Blood Pressure
The Bible Cure for Memory Loss
The Bible Cure for Menopause
The Bible Cure for Osteoporosis
The Bible Cure for PMS and Mood Swings
The Bible Cure for Sleep Disorders
The Bible Cure for Weight Loss and Muscle Gain

SILOAM PRESS
A part of Strang Communications Company
600 Rinehart Road
Lake Mary, FL 34746
(800) 599-5750